AF442588

Table of Contents

Cardio Yoga: Benefits, Guide, and How It Compares

What is cardio yoga?

Rooted in Indian philosophy, yoga focus on poses, breathing techniques, and meditation practices to enhance consciousness and relieve anxiety.

The practice has become increasingly popular throughout the world as a means to relieve stress, improve sleep, boost mental and emotional health, and relieve general low back and neck pain.

While there are many types of yoga, Hatha yoga is the most commonly practiced, referring to any type of yoga that teaches physical postures.

Most yoga classes — ashtanga, vinyasa, and power yoga — are hatha yoga.

While these types of yoga differ in the series, movement, and pace of the physical postures, they generally aren't thought of as cardio or aerobic exercise.

This is because they focus on breathing techniques, body flow, and postures, rather than dynamic movements that ramp up the intensity and elevate your heart rate.

Conversely, cardio yoga workouts involve performing yoga-inspired movements at a quicker pace and with continuous flow to engage more muscles and challenge your cardiovascular, or circulatory, system.

Summary

Unlike traditional yoga, which focuses on breathing techniques, body flow, and postures, cardio yoga incorporates more dynamic movements that ramp up the intensity and elevate your heart rate.

Specific cardio yoga workouts

Because there's not an accepted definition of cardio yoga, instructors may mix in their own favorite movements and movement sequences.

While yoga is generally safe, make sure you're on a flat surface and don't have any conditions that may interfere with balance, such as neuropathy or orthopedic-related limitations.

Here are a few moderate-intensity cardio yoga workouts to try that work all your major muscle groups, including your arms, chest, back, and legs.

Surya Namaskar (Sun Salutation)

Surya Namaskar, commonly known as the Sun Salutation, is a series of postures performed in a sequence.

Here is the sequence:

1. **Samasthiti.** Start standing up straight with your feet together and weight evenly distributed. Your shoulders should be rolled back and

your hands should be hanging by your side with your chin parallel to the ground.

2. Urdhva hastasana. Inhale and bend your knees slightly, raising your arms over your head. Bring your palms together and look at your thumbs.

3. Uttanasana. Exhale and straighten your legs. Bend forward from the hips and bring your hands down. Relax your neck.

4. Urdvah uttanasana. Inhale and lengthen your spine, looking forward and opening your shoulders.

5. Chaturanga dandasana. Exhale and jump or step your feet back. Bend your elbows and keep them tucked into your sides. Lower your body. You may either keep your knees off the floor, or modify the exercise by bringing your knees to the ground.

6. Urdhva mukha svanasana. Inhale and point your toes away from your body. Lift your chest while your knees stay off the ground. Open your shoulders and look up to the sky.

7. Adho mukha svanasana. Exhale and tuck your toes under, lifting your hips and bringing your shoulders down. Look at your navel. You may wish to stay in this position for up to five deep breaths.

8. Urdhva uttanasana. Inhale and jump or step your feet together between your hands, lengthen the spine and look to the front while opening your shoulders (same as step 4).

9. Uttanasana. Exhale and lower the crown of your head toward the ground and relax your neck (same as step 3).

10. Urdhva hastasana. Inhale and bend your knees, raising your arms over your head and bringing your palms together while looking at your thumbs (same as step 2).

11. Samasthiti. Exhale and straighten your legs, bringing your arms to your sides (same as step 1).

Complete this sequence at a relatively quick pace and repeat it for 20 minutes with no rest in between to keep your heart rate elevated.

Other movements

Here are other movements that you can do as part of a sequence:

• **Child's pose pushup.** Starting in a kneeling plank position, perform a kneeling pushup then sit back onto your heels with your arms extended in front (child's pose). Bring your body forward into the kneeling plank position and repeat.

• **Leg lift pigeon sequence.** Starting in plank pose, slightly lift your hips as you raise your left leg toward the ceiling. Slowly pull the left leg back down and through, tucking your knee in toward your chest. Lift your left leg again toward the ceiling, and this time as you pull your left knee through, allow the outer portion of your left leg to rest on the floor as you lower your left glute down. Return to the starting position and repeat with your right let.

- **Walk downs.** Starting from a standing position, bend at the hips and walk yourself down to a plank position. Push yourself into downward facing dog by pushing your hips to the sky. Hold this position for 1–2 seconds. Slowly walk yourself back, maintaining hand contact with the floor. Return to the standing position and repeat.

Perform each movement 10–15 times before moving onto the next exercise.

You can separate these movements with 30-second activities like jumping jacks, air squats, and stationary lunges to keep your body moving and heart rate elevated.

Summary

These cardio yoga workouts are of moderate aerobic intensity and utilize all the major muscle groups.

Weight loss

Although yoga has been suggested to aid weight loss, studies have found conflicting results.

A review of 30 studies including over 2,000 participants found that yoga did not affect weight, body mass index (BMI), waist circumference, or body fat percentage.

However, when the researchers analyzed studies in people with overweight or obesity, yoga was found to significantly reduce BMI.

Still, some variables, such as different types of bias among the studies, may have influenced the study results.

In either case, while beginner to intermediate-level yoga sessions aren't typically considered adequate for improving cardiovascular fitness, more intensive forms of yoga like cardio yoga can train your heart while increasing calories burned and aiding weight loss.

That said, performing cardio yoga at least 5 times per week for 30 minutes may help you lose weight, if that's your goal.

However, keep in mind that exercise alone is rarely enough to lose a significant amount of weight and keep it off — you must also consume fewer calories than you burn.

Generally, reducing your daily calorie intake by 500 is sufficient for weight loss.

You can estimate your calorie needs by using a calorie needs calculator.

Summary

Performing cardio yoga can ramp up calorie burning and aid weight loss in combination with a low calorie diet.

Comparison with other cardio exercises

The metabolic equivalent of task (MET) is one measure researchers use to estimate how many calories are burned during an activity.

One MET represents the number of calories you burn at rest based on the amount of oxygen you consume.

An exercise that is 3 METs requires you to use approximately three times the oxygen compared with 1 MET (at rest), meaning it requires more energy and burns more calories.

A review of 17 studies demonstrated that the METs of yoga ranges from 2 METs during a basic yoga class to 6 METs with Surya Namaskar for an average of 2.9 METs.

For comparison, here are the METs of common forms of cardio:

- walking, moderate pace: 4.8 METs

- elliptical, moderate effort: 5 METs

- jogging, average pace: 7 METs

- biking, average pace: 7 METs

- hiking: 7.8 METs

- stair climbing, fast pace: 8.8 METs

- running, average pace: 9.8 METs

Based on the MET values, yoga at 2.9 METs significantly underperforms when it comes to energy usage and therefore calories burned.

However, at 6 METs, Surya Namaskar and other yoga-inspired cardio workouts may be comparable to exercising on an elliptical at a moderate effort but less intense than jogging at an average pace in regards to calories burned.

Interestingly, Surya Namaskar may not only increase calories burned but also help build muscle.

In one study, participants performed 24 cycles of Surya Namaskar, 6 days a week for 6 months.

At the end of the study, participants demonstrated increased muscle strength when performing bench and shoulder press exercises.

However, the study lacked a control group, which prevents a cause and effect relationship.

Additional studies are necessary to determine whether yoga or more intense cardio yoga workouts can increase muscle strength or size.

Summary

More intense versions of yoga like cardio yoga burn a similar number of calories as exercising on an elliptical at a moderate effort but fewer calories than jogging.

The bottom line

Cardio yoga is a more intense version of traditional yoga, which is generally not thought of as cardio.

It combines yoga-inspired and dynamic movements in various sequences to increase and sustain an elevated heart rate, helping train your heart and burn calories.

Cardio yoga outperforms walking at a moderate pace or exercising on an elliptical at a moderate effort — but not jogging, hiking, or running — in regards to calories burned.

13 Benefits of Yoga That Are Supported by Science

Derived from the Sanskrit word "yuji," meaning yoke or union, yoga is an ancient practice that brings together mind and body.

It incorporates breathing exercises, meditation and poses designed to encourage relaxation and reduce stress.

Practicing yoga is said to come with many benefits for both mental and physical health, though not all of these benefits have been backed by science.

This article takes a look at 13 evidence-based benefits of yoga.

1. Can Decrease Stress

Yoga is known for its ability to ease stress and promote relaxation.

In fact, multiple studies have shown that it can decrease the secretion of cortisol, the primary stress hormone.

One study demonstrated the powerful effect of yoga on stress by following 24 women who perceived themselves as emotionally distressed.

After a three-month yoga program, the women had significantly lower levels of cortisol. They also had lower levels of stress, anxiety, fatigue and depression.

Another study of 131 people had similar results, showing that 10 weeks of yoga helped reduce stress and anxiety. It also helped improve quality of life and mental health.

When used alone or along with other methods of alleviating stress, such as meditation, yoga can be a powerful way to keep stress in check.

Summary: Studies show that yoga can help ease stress and lower your levels of the stress hormone cortisol.

2. Relieves Anxiety

Many people begin practicing yoga as a way to cope with feelings of anxiety.

Interestingly enough, there is quite a bit of research showing that yoga can help reduce anxiety.

In one study, 34 women diagnosed with an anxiety disorder participated in yoga classes twice weekly for two months.

At the end of the study, those who practiced yoga had significantly lower levels of anxiety than the control group.

Another study followed 64 women with post-traumatic stress disorder (PTSD), which is characterized by severe anxiety and fear following exposure to a traumatic event.

After 10 weeks, the women who practiced yoga once weekly had fewer symptoms of PTSD. In fact, 52% of participants no longer met the criteria for PTSD at all.

It's not entirely clear exactly how yoga is able to reduce symptoms of anxiety. However, it emphasizes the importance of being present in the moment and finding a sense of peace, which could help treat anxiety.

Summary: Several studies show that practicing yoga can lead to a decrease in symptoms of anxiety.

3. May Reduce Inflammation

In addition to improving your mental health, some studies suggest that practicing yoga may reduce inflammation as well.

Inflammation is a normal immune response, but chronic inflammation can contribute to the development of pro-inflammatory diseases, such as heart disease, diabetes and cancer.

A 2015 study divided 218 participants into two groups: those who practiced yoga regularly and those who didn't. Both groups then performed moderate and strenuous exercises to induce stress.

At the end of the study, the individuals who practiced yoga had lower levels of inflammatory markers than those who didn't.

Similarly, a small 2014 study showed that 12 weeks of yoga reduced inflammatory markers in breast cancer survivors with persistent fatigue.

Although more research is needed to confirm the beneficial effects of yoga on inflammation, these findings indicate that it may help protect against certain diseases caused by chronic inflammation.

Summary: Some studies show that yoga may reduce inflammatory markers in the body and help prevent pro-inflammatory diseases.

4. Could Improve Heart Health

From pumping blood throughout the body to supplying tissues with important nutrients, the health of your heart is an essential component of overall health.

Studies show that yoga may help improve heart health and reduce several risk factors for heart disease.

One study found that participants over 40 years of age who practiced yoga for five years had a lower blood pressure and pulse rate than those who didn't.

High blood pressure is one of the major causes of heart problems, such as heart attacks and stroke. Lowering your blood pressure can help reduce the risk of these problems.

Some research also suggests that incorporating yoga into a healthy lifestyle could help slow the progression of heart disease.

A study followed 113 patients with heart disease, looking at the effects of a lifestyle change that included one year of yoga training combined with dietary modifications and stress management.

Participants saw a 23% decrease in total cholesterol and a 26% reduction in "bad" LDL cholesterol. Additionally, the progression of heart disease stopped in 47% of patients.

It's unclear how much of a role yoga may have had versus other factors like diet. Yet it can minimize stress, one of the major contributors to heart disease.

Summary: Alone or in combination with a healthy lifestyle, yoga may help decrease risk factors for heart disease.

5. Improves Quality of Life

Yoga is becoming increasingly common as an adjunct therapy to improve quality of life for many individuals.

In one study, 135 seniors were assigned to either six months of yoga, walking or a control group. Practicing yoga significantly improved quality of life, as well as mood and fatigue, compared to the other groups.

Other studies have looked at how yoga can improve quality of life and reduce symptoms in patients with cancer.

One study followed women with breast cancer undergoing chemotherapy. Yoga decreased symptoms of chemotherapy, such as nausea and vomiting, while also improving overall quality of life.

A similar study looked at how eight weeks of yoga affected women with breast cancer. At the end of the study, the women had less pain and fatigue with improvements in levels of invigoration, acceptance and relaxation.

Other studies have found that yoga may help improve sleep quality, enhance spiritual well-being, improve social function and reduce symptoms of anxiety and depression in patients with cancer.

Summary: Some studies show that yoga could improve quality of life and may be used as an adjunct therapy for some conditions.

6. May Fight Depression

Some studies show that yoga may have an anti-depressant effect and could help decrease symptoms of depression.

This may be because yoga is able to decrease levels of cortisol, a stress hormone that influences levels of serotonin, the neurotransmitter often associated with depression.

In one study, participants in an alcohol dependence program practiced Sudarshan Kriya, a specific type of yoga that focuses on rhythmic breathing.

After two weeks, participants had fewer symptoms of depression and lower levels of cortisol. They also had lower levels of ACTH, a hormone responsible for stimulating the release of cortisol.

Other studies have had similar results, showing an association between practicing yoga and decreased symptoms of depression.

Based on these results, yoga may help fight depression, alone or in combination with traditional methods of treatment.

Summary: Several studies have found that yoga may decrease symptoms of depression by influencing the production of stress hormones in the body.

7. Could Reduce Chronic Pain

Chronic pain is a persistent problem that affects millions of people and has a range of possible causes, from injuries to arthritis.

There is a growing body of research demonstrating that practicing yoga could help reduce many types of chronic pain.

In one study, 42 individuals with carpal tunnel syndrome either received a wrist splint or did yoga for eight weeks.

At the end of the study, yoga was found to be more effective in reducing pain and improving grip strength than wrist splinting.

Another study in 2005 showed that yoga could help decrease pain and improve physical function in participants with osteoarthritis of the knees.

Although more research is needed, incorporating yoga into your daily routine may be beneficial for those who suffer from chronic pain.

Summary: Yoga may help reduce chronic pain in conditions like carpal tunnel syndrome and osteoarthritis.

8. Could Promote Sleep Quality

Poor sleep quality has been associated with obesity, high blood pressure and depression, among other disorders.

Studies show that incorporating yoga into your routine could help promote better sleep.

In a 2005 study, 69 elderly patients were assigned to either practice yoga, take an herbal preparation or be part of the control group.

The yoga group fell asleep faster, slept longer and felt more well-rested in the morning than the other groups.

Another study looked at the effects of yoga on sleep in patients with lymphoma. They found that it decreased sleep disturbances, improved sleep quality and duration and reduced the need for sleep medications.

Though the way it works is not clear, yoga has been shown to increase the secretion of melatonin, a hormone that regulates sleep and wakefulness.

Yoga also has a significant effect on anxiety, depression, chronic pain and stress — all common contributors to sleep problems.

Summary: Yoga may help enhance sleep quality because of its effects on melatonin and its impact on several common contributors to sleep problems.

9. Improves Flexibility and Balance

Many people add yoga to their fitness routine to improve flexibility and balance.

There is considerable research that backs this benefit, demonstrating that it can optimize performance through the use of specific poses that target flexibility and balance.

A recent study looked at the impact of 10 weeks of yoga on 26 male college athletes. Doing yoga significantly increased several measures of flexibility and balance, compared to the control group.

Another study assigned 66 elderly participants to either practice yoga or calisthenics, a type of body weight exercise.

After one year, total flexibility of the yoga group increased by nearly four times that of the calisthenics group.

A 2013 study also found that practicing yoga could help improve balance and mobility in older adults.

Practicing just 15–30 minutes of yoga each day could make a big difference for those looking to enhance performance by increasing flexibility and balance.

Summary: Research shows that practicing yoga can help improve balance and increase flexibility.

10. Could Help Improve Breathing

Pranayama, or yogic breathing, is a practice in yoga that focuses on controlling the breath through breathing exercises and techniques.

Most types of yoga incorporate these breathing exercises, and several studies have found that practicing yoga could help improve breathing.

In one study, 287 college students took a 15-week class where they were taught various yoga poses and breathing exercises. At the end of the study, they had a significant increase in vital capacity.

Vital capacity is a measure of the maximum amount of air that can be expelled from the lungs. It is especially important for those with lung disease, heart problems and asthma.

Another study in 2009 found that practicing yogic breathing improved symptoms and lung function in patients with mild-to-moderate asthma.

Improving breathing can help build endurance, optimize performance and keep your lungs and heart healthy.

Summary: Yoga incorporates many breathing exercises, which could help improve breathing and lung function.

11. May Relieve Migraines

Migraines are severe recurring headaches that affect an estimated 1 out of 7 Americans each year.

Traditionally, migraines are treated with medications to relieve and manage symptoms.

However, increasing evidence shows that yoga could be a useful adjunct therapy to help reduce migraine frequency.

A 2007 study divided 72 patients with migraines into either a yoga therapy or self-care group for three months.

Practicing yoga led to reductions in headache intensity, frequency and pain compared to the self-care group.

Another study treated 60 patients with migraines using conventional care with or without yoga. Doing yoga resulted in a greater decrease in headache frequency and intensity than conventional care alone.

Researchers suggest that doing yoga may help stimulate the vagus nerve, which has been shown to be effective in relieving migraines.

Summary: Studies show that yoga may stimulate the vagus nerve and reduce migraine intensity and frequency, alone or in combination with conventional care.

12. Promotes Healthy Eating Habits

Mindful eating, also known as intuitive eating, is a concept that encourages being present in the moment while eating.

It's about paying attention to the taste, smell and texture of your food and noticing any thoughts, feelings or sensations you experience while eating.

This practice has been shown to promote healthy eating habits that help control blood sugar, increase weight loss and treat disordered eating behaviors.

Because yoga places a similar emphasis on mindfulness, some studies show that it could be used to encourage healthy eating behaviors.

One study incorporated yoga into an outpatient eating disorder treatment program with 54 patients, finding that yoga helped reduce both eating disorder symptoms and preoccupation with food.

Another small study looked at how yoga affected symptoms of binge eating disorder, a disorder characterized by compulsive overeating and a feeling of loss of control.

Yoga was found to cause a decrease in episodes of binge eating, an increase in physical activity and a small decrease in weight.

For those with and without disordered eating behaviors, practicing mindfulness through yoga can aid in the development of healthy eating habits.

Summary: Yoga encourages mindfulness, which may be used to help promote mindful eating and healthy eating habits.

13. Can Increase Strength

In addition to improving flexibility, yoga is a great addition to an exercise routine for its strength-building benefits.

In fact, there are specific poses in yoga that are designed to increase strength and build muscle.

In one study, 79 adults performed 24 cycles of sun salutations — a series of foundational poses often used as a warm-up — six days a week for 24 weeks.

They experienced a significant increase in upper body strength, endurance and weight loss. Women had a decrease in body fat percentage, as well.

A 2015 study had similar findings, showing that 12 weeks of practice led to improvements in endurance, strength and flexibility in 173 participants.

Based on these findings, practicing yoga can be an effective way to boost strength and endurance, especially when used in combination with a regular exercise routine.

Summary: Some studies show that yoga can cause an increase in strength, endurance and flexibility.

The Bottom Line

Multiple studies have confirmed the many mental and physical benefits of yoga.

Incorporating it into your routine can help enhance your health, increase strength and flexibility and reduce symptoms of stress, depression and anxiety.

Finding the time to practice yoga just a few times per week may be enough to make a noticeable difference when it comes to your health.